Essential Oils: Aromatherapy

A Complete Guide of Essential Oils And Aromatherapy

I0439775

Hanna Krem is a world-class chef and health expert that has setup meal plans and diets for hundreds of thousands of people across the world. As a bonus for purchasing her book, she has added a bonus of the world's BEST super fruits and vegetables that you must eat to gain OPTIMAL health.

To receive the free gift, visit **www.strengthrecipe.com/free**

Disclaimer

Summary

Essential oils have been around for many years although they have been modified time and again in line with advancement in technology. However, more and more people are discovering their amazing benefits today and you can be one of them.

In this book, we'll look at what essential oils are in to give you a background on it. After that we'll move on to the advantages and disadvantages of these essential oils then to the advantages and disadvantages of perennial vegetables. If you have been wondering about the different recipes for essential oils that help you relax, reduce stress and stimulate mental health then you are lucky because we are tackling that too. Generally, we'll provide you with the facts you need to know about essential oils.

Table of Contents

Introduction

There might be a lot of talk around you regarding essential oils and you are wondering what kinds of oils they might be. An essential oil is simply a liquid distilled from the flowers, leaves, roots, stems, bark and various elements of a plant. Most of the time, water or steam is used to distill these liquids. You may think that these essential oils have elements of oil in them due to the word "oil" but this is not the case.

Most of the essential oils are clear in color although there are oils like orange, lemongrass and patchouli that can either have the yellow or amber color. Essential oils carry the true essence of the particular plants they are derived from. They are normally confused with perfume or fragrance oils yet they are quite different. Essential oils are created from true plants while perfume oils are derived from artificially created fragrances. The perfumes do not have the therapeutic benefits of essential oils.

There are various methods in which you can get the therapeutic benefits of essential oils. Examples include inhaling them or applying them directly on the skin. You can buy the various essential oils because they offer different benefits. The great thing about essential oils is that you can blend them together to be able to get all the different benefits at once. You can also purchase essential oils that have already been blended. The only disadvantage is that you have no control over the blending process and so you just have to do with the oils included.

Chapter 1: Benefits of essential oils

Essential oils contain numerous benefits and we are going to look at some of them.

1.   Are able to penetrate your skin immediately

One of the benefits of essential oils is the fact that they are able to penetrate through your skin and cell membranes immediately. It only takes seconds for them to diffuse through your blood and tissues. These oils have the ability to get through the brain-blood barrier in order to get to the amygdale and various limbic parts of the brain. These are the parts that are in charge of controlling our mood, beliefs and emotions. This means that essential oils are capable of changing these three in order to enable us cope with stress, anger and the various emotions we are facing.

2.   They have oxygenating properties

Essential oils contain oxygen molecules. They can therefore transport this oxygen to other cells in our bodies that are deprived of oxygen and to cells that need nutrients too. The cells in our body need oxygen to be healthy in order to be able to perform their functions properly and essential oils help with this.

3.   They soothe muscles and joints

If you are suffering from aching muscles and joints then essential oils might be a good remedy for that. You may have minor aches and pains due to the everyday activities you engage in and essential oils can still help to take care of this. When you combine them with massage then you get even better results.

4.   They contain high levels of antioxidants

Essential oils have been known to contain high level of antioxidants, which help the body. Antioxidants are responsible for strengthening your body's system. This enables the body to prevent negative effects that diet, aging and the environment have on our bodies. They also do away with free radicals. If you want to know the antioxidant capacity that essential oil contain then look at the ORAC (Oxygen Radical Absorbance Capacity) value indicated. For example clove essential oil's ORAC value is 1, 078, 700 µTE/100g. This is very high compared to the one for carrots, which is at 210 µTE/100g.

5.   They soothe digestion

Essential oils have been known to soothe digestion. Peppermints also known as *Mentha Piperita* are great herbs known for soothing digestions. They can also help to restore your digestive efficiency.

6.   Are convenient and easy to use.

Essential oils are quite convenient in the sense that you can use them anywhere. Did you know that you could wear essential oils during the day? Yes, it is true and you can do this whether you are at home or work place. You can even carry them in your pocket. These oils are important in massage too and they can improve your level of meditation and concentration.

7.   Can be used on animals too

It's amazing that the use of essential oils is not limited to humans. Animals have been known to respond well to these oils too and great examples are dogs and horses. Although there are some limitations when it comes to cats, they can still be used on them.

8.   Are safe for use

Essential oils have the ability to restore your body's balance without harming it. This is due to the fact that they do not contain any chemical based products. However, ensure to choose therapeutic grade essential oils and not the perfume grade ones because the latter are made of up harmful chemicals.

9.   Multi –purpose

There are essential oils that perform more than one function. For example, true lavender essential oil also known, as *Lavandula angustifolia* is great for cuts and minor burns because it is gentle on the skin and contains antimicrobial properties too. It can also promote sleep and relaxation when inhaled. Therefore you don't need to buy lots of essential oils.

10.   Essential oils refine your skin

Using beauty products with lots of chemicals can sometimes diminish your natural glow. However, when you resort to essential oils then you can have it back. Essential oils help to give you a clear-looking complexion. In addition to that, they reduce the appearance of aging signs and give you healthy-looking hair.

11.   Create deep spiritual awareness

Essential oils have always been used in both spiritual and religious ceremonies. They help people to connect with a higher being than themselves. According to research, these essential oils have compounds that stimulate olfactory receptors. If you want to enhance your spiritual experience then you can dilute the essential oils and apply them directly to your feet, wrists, behind the ears or let them diffuse in a quiet environment where you want to have your spiritual meditation.

Chapter 2: How to choose and use essential oils

You may know about the benefits you stand to gain from essential oils but have no idea how to begin using them. Do not worry because this essential oils guide to will help you figure out how to choose and then use essential oils.

What you have to know about essential oils before you buy them is that they serve different purposes and so you should make your choice based on what function you would like it to perform. For example there are essential oils responsible for treating burns, elevating your mood and so on. It is important to find out more about the different essential oils and how you can identify the one you need. A good place to start is by reading. There are essential oils books available that can help you find the particular essential oil suitable for your particular need. While doing this, it is important to read about the cautions provided for each essential oil and the methods of application. We are going to look at some examples although it is quite important to dilute the oils as instructed. Monitor your reaction to these oils and watch out for any adverse effects.

There are many questions that people normally ask about essential oils to give them a better understanding of what they entail and how to use them.

How should I use the essential oils?

There are three ways in which essential oils can get in to your body. You can inhale them, apply them on your skin or ingest them. These three ways are broken down into many kinds of methods used to apply them. For example, you can use spray, compresses, massage or baths to apply them on your skin.

How should I choose a method of application?

We've already established that there are many methods of application and you may wonder how to choose the most suitable one for you. There are factors you need to consider to help you make this choice and they are, the type of essential oil you want to use and the desired effect you hope to achieve. For example, wound care requires topical applications most of the time; baths need both topical absorption and inhalation while inhalation and topical application are recommended for mood effects. In case you are not sure of the application method you should use then it is advisable to consult an experienced aroma therapist.

How should I go about inhaling the essential oils?

There are various devices and techniques used to inhale essential oils.

➢ Diffuser

Essential oils are normally placed inside the diffuser. Water may be added too and even heat to help it evaporate. However, it is important to read the instructions first, don't just include the water and heat automatically. If you are advised to put it under heat, it is important to knot that essential oils should not be subjected to direct heat because this will change their chemical structure. Diffusers are different and there are some with timers for convenience. Get instructions on how to use the one you have.

➢ Dry evaporation

Put several drops of the essential oil on a piece of tissue or cotton ball and let it evaporate in to the air. If your aim is to get an intense dose of the essential oils then you can try sniffing the cotton ball. If your aim is a milder dose then you can have the cotton within your vicinity. For example, you can put it on your desk when you are on your computer.

➢ Steam

Add some drops of the essential oil you are using in a bowl of steaming water. This will make the oil to vaporize. Cover your head and the bowl of water using a towel and breathe deeply.

z

Try not to use more than 2 drops of the essential oils because this method is quite direct and too much of it ight be overwhelming. Make sure you keep your eyes closed during this method. This method is not recommended for children below 7 years old. Children above 7 years who need to use this method should cover their eyes with swimming goggles for protection purposes.

➢ **Spray.** Put drops of the essential oils inside a water-based solution. Shake it and then spray in the air in order to set a good mood and deodorize the room. For example, if you want to portray the holiday feeling in a room then you can use a solution of citrus oils to do this. Ensure you shake the bottle before you spray it to avoid a situation where you spray the water and not the solution, which might have settled at the bottom.

How are essentially oils applied topically?

There are a variety of techniques that can be used to apply essential oils topically. What you should have at the back of your mind is that most of the essential oils, are not meant to be directly applied to your skin. That is why they are normally diluted first.

How are solutions prepared?

The rule of preparing solutions is that you should always dilute essential oils in a carrier substance. Examples of the carrier substances you can use include water or nut or vegetable oil. Their concentration shouldn't be more than 3-5%. When using the solution for massage or when you want to apply it over large sections of your body then a 1% solution is recommended. This is about a drop of the essential oil in case you are using one teaspoon of carrier. 0.25% is enough for infants and 0.5% for toddlers. It is important to shake the solution in this case too before applying it.

Which carrier oils are suitable?

It is easy to get common carrier oils in stores that sell natural body and bath products. There are even natural food stores that have them. However, cold-pressed and organic oils are recommended and examples of these include apricot kernel, jojoba oil, almond oil, avocado oil and grape-seed oil. These oils have a mild smell of their own. These oils should be refrigerated until when you want to use them. In case you notice any rancid smell from them then you should throw them away. They can stay for about a year when refrigerated before giving of the bad smell.

What are the techniques?

➢ **Compress.** The first step is diluting the essential oil in a liquid carrier (you can choose oil or water) before being applied directly to the affected place or to a dressing. You can apply heat or cold.

An example includes adding some drops of ginger essential oil to hot water and mixing it. You can soak a piece of cloth inside the mixture and put on your stiff joint. You can apply some heat if you wish.

➢ **Gargle.** Add drops of essential oil to the water and then mix it before gargling the solution. Make sure you do not swallow it, spit it out instead. You can do this if you are having a sore throat and tea tree oil is great for this purpose.

> **Bath.**

Add drops of essential oils to your bath water, which is in a dispersant. Step in to the bath water. Your skin will be able to absorb these oils and inhale the volatilized essential oil. Full cream milk can act as a dispersant and a few tablespoons are enough. When doing this, keep in mind that essential oils will float on the bath water because they are not water-soluble. You will able to capture the full strength of the essential oils when you pass through them. Bath salts can also disperse essential oils. You can use one part, two parts and three parts of baking soda, Epsom salts and sea salt respectively to come up with a relaxing bath base. Mix together this solution and true lavender essential oil in a ratio of 2 to 6 tablespoons and drops respectively. Mix it with your bath water and get in.

> **Massage.** Choose natural carrier oils and add drops of essential oil to it. Rub it

gently on your skin. Stick to the same quantity mentioned in the introduction of "how solutions are prepared".

How are oils applied internally?

There is internal application of essential oils and this can be done in various ways. Examples include suppositories and oral ingestion. However, you have to know that this method is only allowed in the U.S when supervised by a licensed healthcare provider.

Chapter 3: Essential Oil recipes for relaxation and stress relief

Stress has been proven to be one of the leading causes of many health problems and even deaths in extreme cases. The life we live today exposes us to higher risks of stress and this is why there has been an increase in the number of people looking for stress remedies. There are various methods used by different people to deal with stress and using essential oils is one of them.

Essential oils are known to give you a relaxing and calming effect, which we need in our busy lives. The essential oils do this with the use of aromatherapy.

There are some home remedies that you may use to create that happy and calming effect. You may wonder how aromatherapy is connected to stress reduction. Well, it stimulates limbic and endocrine systems and these are the systems responsible for your hormones and emotions. When this happens, it triggers both an emotional and physical response, which is positive in this case. An example is what happens if you happen to smell Lavender essential oil. The microscopic chemicals in it trigger your system, which responds by calming down your nervous system leading to relaxing of muscles.

There have been several studies conducted on the link between aromatherapy and stress reduction and the results were positive. It was discovered that people suffering from Alzheimer's disease were treated with lemon and lavender essential oils and this reduced their level of agitation. Depressed men took less anti-depressant after using citrus essential oils. Ylang ylang essential oils were discovered to boost the production of endorphins in the body and these are the hormones responsible for reducing pain and giving you the feeling of being well. All these prove that aromatherapy works for stress reduction and relaxation.

Examples of the best essential oils to help you reduce stress and tension include lavender, marjoram, benzoin, geranium, Melissa, vanilla, orange, cinnamon, neroli, rose, ylang ylang and chamomile among others.

Strategies for aromatherapy stress relief

I know that you've told over and over again to take good care of yourself but I have to say it again. Self-care is essential in helping your body fight stress. Most of us say that we would like to take better care of ourselves but we don't have the time. However, when you really think about it, it will cost you more in terms of time and money if you don't take care of yourself. Just stop doing too much. If you start to feel out of control then you can take small breaks during the day to calm yourself down. Doing this twice a day for about 5 minutes is enough. You can increase this amount of time later on to about 15 minutes when your tolerance level increases. If you find this difficult then you can try using the aromatherapy inhaler recipe.

Making your own aromatherapy inhaler

Having your own aromatherapy inhaler is great because it is quite portable. You can therefore have it with you all the time because it is small and can fit in your bag, car and therefore can use it whenever need arises.

Ingredients

- 1 teaspoon of coarse sea salt.
- 10 Drops of Bergamot essential oil.
- 4 Drops of Orange essential oil.
- 4 Drops of Lavender essential oil.
- 1 Drop of Chamomile or Ylang ylang essential oil.
- 1 Drop of Rose Geranium essential oil.
- Glass bottles.

Procedure

1. Pour the coarse sea salt inside an extremely small and dark plastic bottle or glass.
2. Add all the other ingredients to it.
3. Inhale the aroma in three slow deep breaths.
4. Relax for a while and inhale the aroma again in three deep breaths. Ensure you do this thrice and you will have great aromatherapy stress relief.

Scented mineral bath of
Ylang ylang and lemon

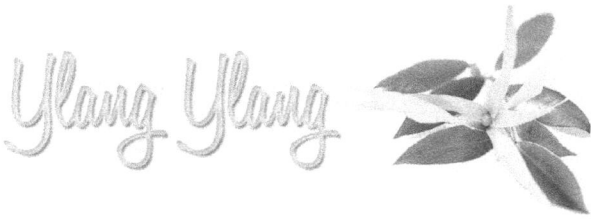

These essential oils are great for your senses. They are great because they are moderately relaxing and energizing and have a clean sweet fragrance.

Ingredients

- 1 tablespoon of baking soda.
- 2 tablespoons of sea salt.
- 1-½ teaspoons of borax.
- 6 Drops of lemon essential oils.
- 4 Drops of ylang ylang.
-

Procedure

1.   Mix together the baking soda, sea salt, and borax.

2. Add the lemon and ylang ylang essential oils to the mixture and mix well.

3. Prepare a bath and pour the mixture inside under running water. Ensure the salts completely dissolve and the oils evenly dispersed in the water. You can add some drops of Lavender to create a good balance.

Lavender, Chamomile and Tangerine blend

This blend is great for relaxation and stress reduction. It will make your muscles, tissues and joints relax and give you a good energy balance.

Ingredients

- 3 Drops of Tangerine.
- 3 Drops of Lavender.
- 3 Drops of Chamomile.
- 1 ounce of carrier oil. (Choose any)

Procedure

1. Blend the above essential oils together inside the carrier oil.
2. Massage as desired.

This blend can also act as bath oil.

Rose Otto

This aroma is quite an effective aphrodisiac. It has benefits on both your mind and body. It has the ability to relax your spirit and relieve you of stress. You can enjoy it as a relaxing bath.

Ingredients

- Bath water.
- 3 ½ tablespoons of heavy cream.
- 3 Drops of the Turkish Rose-Otto essential oil.

Procedure

1.   Mix the heavy cream and Turkish Rose-Otto essential oil.

2. Add the mixture to the bath water.

3. Get in to your bath water and enjoy.

If you want a more sensuous scent then you can add some drops of Jasmine or Sandalwood essential oils.

Tension taming recipes

This aromatherapy bath salt recipe will help to ease away your tension. They do this by balancing your nervous system which affects your mood swings too. This recipe is quite good especially for those with oily skin because it helps to cleanse the skin and reduce the production of oil in addition to healing blemished skin.

Ingredients

- 1 cup of sea salt.
- 3 Drops of the Lavender essential oil.
- 6 Drops of Bergamot essential oil.
- ½ cup of baking soda.
- 6 Drops of the sweet Orange essential oil.
- 4 Drops of yellow and 6 drops of red food coloring. (This is optional)

Procedure

1.   Use a metal spoon to mix together the salt and baking soda. (A metal spoon is recommended because a wooden spoon will be ruined from absorbing the essential oils).

2. Pour drops of the essential oils on top of the salts and stir it until it is properly mixed. Do the same with the food coloring.

3. Keep the mixture inside a plastic jar or dark glass and leave it for 24 hours before using it.

4. A cup of salt is enough for a single bath. This recipe you just made can last for three baths.

It is important to note that sweet orange and Bergamot should not be used before being exposed to the sun. This is due to the fact that they have the ability to cause sunburn and photosensitivity.

Aromatherapy bath oil recipe for relaxing

This recipe for bath oil is super relaxing and it will make you very calm and at peace. All you need to do is take some slow, deep breaths of it and all your stress will melt away. The deep scent of this bath oil is especially great for men. You can use it as massage oil for your man and this will help him relax to an extent that he might even fall asleep. Sandal wood essential oil is part of the ingredients used for this bath oil and it is important for healing the skin. Therefore if you have skin conditions such as psoriasis and eczema then this bath oil is good for you. In addition to that, it helps to slow down the aging process and revitalizes your skin.

Ingredients

- 12 Drops of the Lavender essential oil.
- 4fl oz. equivalent of 125 ml of the carrier oil you prefer. Examples include almond and jojoba oil.
- 30 Drops of the Sandalwood essential oil.
- 2 Drops of Cedar wood essential oil.

Procedure

1.　　　　Mix all the ingredients together inside a plastic bottle or dark glass. Store the bottle inside a cool, dark place. (Keep it away from your bathroom because of the warmth and humidity)

2.　　　　Pour a tablespoon of the aromatherapy bath oil you made in to the bath running after running it. It is as simple as that and you are ready to take that super-relaxing bath that will relieve your stress.

Be careful to avoid going for cheap Sandalwood because it will not give you the same results as the original one. It may be a bit expensive but it is worth your money.

Aromatherapy bath oil for sweet dreams

This bath recipe is quite soothing and is especially good for people suffering from insomnia. This is because it will soothe you to sleep. If you are having one of those days where sleep is elusive then there is no need to worry. You can try out this bath oil, which will calm your nerves and relax your muscles. You will then be able to have a peaceful sleep when your mind is calm too. In addition to that, the essential oils will help to repair your skin and reduce the appearance of wrinkles. In case you are not able to take a bath then you can massage your face and torso using some of the lavender oil and you will still enjoy its luxurious effect. It is advisable to do this before you get into bed in order to have a deep sleep.

Did you know that you could make your own massage oil? Well, it is possible. Although bath oils are important, you may not always have the time to take a bath. However, if you have the massage oil then you can use it to get the same results. Lavender is pleasing to the eye, has an amazing scent and contains numerous healing powers so preparing Lavender massage oils is a good decision.

This massage oil is great for insomnia, pain, stress and anxiety. When you combine these amazing effects of Lavender with its gentle touch, you are on the right path to achieving an intense kind of relaxation. If you are not in a position to have a full body massage then you can even do some foot massage. This massage oil can also be rubbed on your chest and stomach to help you sleep.

Ingredients

- 2 Drop of the Clary Sage essential oil.
- 12 Drops of the Lavender essential oil.
- 3 Drops of Marjoram essential oil.
- 12 Drops of either Orange or Bergamot essential oil.
- 1 drop of Vetiver essential oil
- ¼ cup of any carrier oil you prefer.

Procedure

1.   Mix all the ingredients together inside a plastic bottle or dark glass. It is advisable to get a bottle or glass with a lotion or oil dispenser cup. This is to avoid accidental spillage.

2.   Wait for a period of 24 hours before using the massage in order to give to time to "cure". The bottle should be stored in a cool, dark place and used within three months.

You can either double or triple the quantity of the ingredients if you want to have a large amount of the massage oil.

One thing you have to remember when choosing carrier oils is that you can tailor them to suit your specific skin needs. It is advisable to choose the ones that help to nourish and support your skin. For example, if you are using jojoba or sweet almond oil then you can add sea buckthorn oil or borage oil to it if you have dry or maturing skin. It is okay to experiment with the different carrier oils in order to find out what suits your skin best. This can be a fun experience.

Chapter 4: Essential oils recipes for mental health

Our mental health is equally as important as our physical health if not more. This is due to the fact that our brain is always working every waking minute and yet it is what holds us together. If we overwork it or subject it to too much stress then we are bound to lose our minds and no one would like that. There are essential oils that are known to improve your mental health. If you want to have a smarter, quicker and clearer brain then essential oils are the way to go. If you open your mind to it, you will be amazed because you can experience the results immediately. These are the five essential oils known to improve your mental clarity.

- Rosemary

- Juniper Berry
- Sage or Clary Sage
- Basil
- Peppermint

There are several ways of using the essential oils to help clear your mind. One of the easiest ways of doing this is by dropping the essential oils inside a pot with lots of water. You can then heat the water until it is steaming before turning down the heat. You can just leave the pot on the burner and the essential oils will evaporate in to the air giving your home the sweet scents of the oil. If you find trouble sleeping at night and you don't want to wake up the whole family by filling the house with essential oils then you can use a candle diffuser. It is as easy as putting the essential oils inside the top bowl before lighting a tea light below it.

The tea light will give off heat, which will make the essential oils evaporate into the air, and you will capture those amazing scents, which will soothe you to sleep.

Rosemary Mist

This will serve to stimulate your senses and is great for after you have showered but just before you towel off. You need to use it when your skin is still damp.

Ingredients

- 6 drops of the rosemary essential oil
- Spray bottle.
- 1 teaspoon of olive oil.
- 5 ounces of distilled water.
- 1 sprig fresh rosemary

Procedure

1.   Add all the ingredients inside the spray bottle and shake well in order for them to mix properly.
2.Spritz it on as you wish.

Alertness massage oil

This massage oil will help to improve your mental health by increasing your brain alertness.

Ingredients

1.   6 Drops of ginger.
2.   4 Drops of Juniper Berry
3.   5 Drops of Grapefruit.
4.   15 ml of your preferred carrier oil.

Procedure

1.   Mix all the ingredients together.
2.   Take drops of it and use it to massage the back of your neck and your temples because it is ready for use.

Mental clarity spray

Mental clarity is part of great mental health and this is the purpose that the spray aims to achieve.

Ingredients

- 50 Drops of lemongrass.
- 20 Drops of Cedarwood
- 40 Drops of Niaouli.
- 40 Drops of rosemary.
- 4 ounces, which is equivalent of 120 ml of pure water.

Procedure

1. Mix together all the essential oils and then add water.
2. Shake well.
3. Put inside the sprayer ready for use whenever you need it.

Alertness spray

When you use this spray, you will be more alert to be able to concentrate on what you are doing.

Ingredients

- 40 Drops of Bergamot
- 25 Drops of Lavender
- 40 Drops of Grapefruit
- 30 Drops of Juniper Berry
- 40 Drops of Peppermint
- 4 ounces of pure water

Procedure

1. Mix all the ingredients together inside a mist sprayer
2. Shake well.
3. Spray it from the mist sprayer.

Refreshing spray

Both our bodies and minds need to be refreshed every now and then to be able to take on more responsibilities.

Ingredients

- 4 oz. of distilled water
- 10 Drops of Orange essential oil
- 5 ml of Emulsifier essential oil
- 50 Drops of lime essential oil
- 50 Drops of Grapefruit essential oil

Procedure

1. Mix together the emulsifier and all the essential oils inside a clean bottle.
2. Add distilled water inside the bottle.
3. Shake the bottle well.
4. Spritz the contents in the air.

Remember to always shake the bottle before you spritz the contents. You can use these ingredients in any diffuser as long as you do away with the water and the emulsifier. You can use an amber bottle to blend it then shake properly before placing some drops in your diffuser.

Blending the various essential oils yourself to serve different purposes is great because you have control over the ingredients you use. However, do not beat yourself up if you don't have the time to make them yourself. You can always buy them. Just ask for the particular essential oils or the blends of essential blends that you need. Either way, you can benefit from them.

Final thoughts

One of the best things about essential oils is the fact that they don't require you to be an aroma therapist in order to benefit from them. Anyone can use them and some come when they are already pre-blended so you don't have to worry about how to go about the process of blending them. What is required of you is simply putting them in a burner or rubbing them on the various pulse joints.

You don't need to have complicated issues to require essential oils. You can use them for something as simple as a burn. Pour cold water on it and use the recommended essential oil such as a mixture of lavender oil and sweet almond oil.

More people are going back to the traditional ways of treatments and preferring natural remedies. This is why the number of people resorting to using essential oils is rising because they can offer the great therapeutic benefits without the worry of the harmful side effects. Try out the essential oils and experience the benefits first hand.

Yours sincerely,
Author.
Hanna M. Krem

Thank you for purchasing and enjoying recipes from Vegetarian Soups: From Around The World: Delicious Vegetarian Soups Under 200 Calories is the perfect cookbook for you. I truly hope you enjoyed cooking with me. This book is the second in a series of Vegetarian Cookbooks that are filled will hundreds of mouthwatering, heart healthy, and family friendly recipes from all over the world.

Please take a moment to leave a review for my book! It is greatly appreciated.

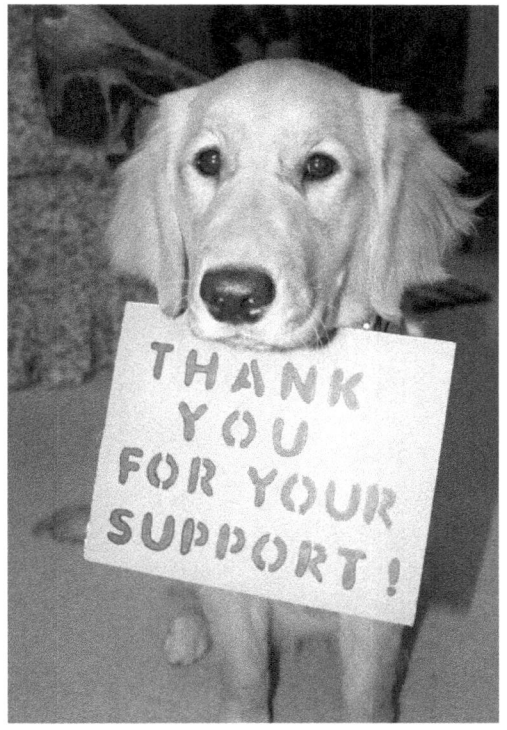

Try my other book below!

Leptin Resistance: Achieve Permanent Weight Loss and Great Health

Seafood Recipes: Ultimate Seafood Soups Under 200 Calories

.